101 WAYS TO LOSE WEIGHT WITHOUT NOTICING.

I0427383

MARIANNE DUVALL.

ISBN: 978 - 1492751960

Contents

Introduction

We seem to spend half our lives on diets nowadays and the other half worrying about it.

And even worse, while we're so concerned about dieting and losing weight, the obesity problem is getting worse and worse each year.

It's a paradox.

Millions of people spending billions of pounds and dollars on diet products and exercise equipment and getting heavier all the time.

Obviously the secret of controlling our weight must be really difficult.

Rubbish!

Losing weight and keeping it off is simple.

Ditch the fad diets.

Avoid the diet food.

Stop feeling like a failure and learn to change your habits one step at a time so that you lose weight and have a healthy lifestyle without noticing.

Losing weight comes in two parts, healthy food choices and more movement. That doesn't mean a starvation diet and half your life at the gym it means small changes that you can live with easily. Little tweaks in your daily routine that you hardly notice that that add up to big results.

Why do so many of us spend our whole lives trying to lose weight, tried to control our eating and trying to do more exercise? And why do we feel a failure season after season, year after year?

Because we think it has to be difficult.

We been brainwashed by the multimillion dollar diet, food and exercise industries to believe that it is terribly difficult, fall too hard for anyone to do on their own. We need their help, their expensive, highly profitable help.

So we need to invest in diet books and buy special foods, we need the DVDs, the exercise equipment and the gym and diet club memberships.

But the sorry fact is that for most of us the only thing that loses weight is our wallet!

The other problem is the mental attitude that this whole industry creates.

It's going to be difficult. We can't possibly do it without all their professional, expert help.

If you start a project, any project expecting it to be difficult that is the mental image you will take into it and you will expect to fail -so you almost certainly will fail.

The other problem is that most of these programs do make it difficult! It's almost as if you are supposed to suffer for carrying a few too many pounds.

It's a sin and you have to be punished you have to struggle to succeed.

So, after a few days of struggle, pain and hunger, you give up. Not worthy of being slim and fit. So why try?

Until another Miracle promise comes along to prise open your wallet.

We are programmed to fail. To endlessly fall for the promises and the hype and then find that we fall short of their expectations. We can't live up to their standards and we end up as failures, consoling ourselves with a tub of ice cream as we sit on the couch.

But the truth is that the programs are designed to make us fail. About 98% of people who start a diet system will end up the same weight or even heavier after a few months. After all, if we succeed, the diet and exercise industry would lose all their profitable customers and they don't want that!

So do yourself a favour. Ditch the latest fad diet, forget the latest fitness miracle and start taking control-one step at a time.

In this book I have concentrated on the food side of losing weight, if you would like some ideas on how to increase your exercise, I have also written *101 ways to exercise without noticing.*

Mindset and weight loss

It is natural to think that losing weight is all about, what you eat and how much you exercise, but actually the most important stage of getting your weight under control is getting the right mental attitude towards your diet.

Successful weight control is not about a lifetime of yoyo dieting, following each new fad, as it hits the bookshelves and the magazines. In fact, that is a sure way to failure.

The road to success begins by you making the decision that you will control your weight and be happy with your weight for the rest of your life.

Once you accept this it will free you from the constant stress of worrying about each pound you might lose or put on.

So as you start this new part of your life, there are some changes you can make to the way you feel about your weight.

1: Think long term. You want to be fit and healthy for the rest of your life, so forget losing a few pounds holiday this and think long-term it's far healthier and will help you make permanent improvements rather than yoyo dieting.

2: Set small realistic goals. Aim to lose 1 or 2lbs a week rather than 10lbs by the weekend.

3: Enjoy the slow but steady successes. The fact that you are constantly winning and reaching each target is far more motivating than starving yourself, losing a dress size and then putting it straight back on the next week.

4: Do the same with fitness. Set small achievable goals so that you can actually reach them and grow your fitness one step at a time.

5: When you've reached your target, enjoy your success and set your next target. In anything that you are trying to do in life, it is far easier to break a task down into small manageable chunks. If you try to face the whole mountain at once you will be overwhelmed by the insurmountable task and you won't have the will to even start. 40 pounds might seem an impossible amount to lose, but 4lbs is much more manageable, so tackle 4lbs 10 times. No matter what your ultimate goal, it will always help if you break it down into small pieces that you can actually imagine succeeding at.

6: Take up a hobby. You often snack because of boredom. If you feel that might be part of your problem, it could help if you find a hobby to occupy your spare time and your hands rather than watching TV with a bowl of snacks and soda. It sounds strange but starting to make jewellery could help you lose weight.

7: Start a money box. This might not seem as if it has anything to do with losing weight, but it has. Find a glass jar or money box, and each time you feel like treating yourself to a full fat latte, a muffin, or a chocolate bar, put the money in the jar instead. It's amazing how much better you'll feel about resisting the fattening treats when you see how much money you are saving.

8: Research has shown that it takes about 30 days to create a new habit, so if you invest 30 minutes a day for 30 days. You can create the new habit that will help you succeed in your goals. For instance, if you decide to go for a swim twice a week before work, and you stick to that for 30 days it will become a habit that you no longer have to think about. The secret of creating new habits is to choose targets that are achievable, rewarding and of course enjoyable, so if you hate swimming that target of swimming twice a week is never going to work, choose something that you will enjoy.

9: Creating a plan is also very important in achieving any target in life. Once you write something down, it becomes more real, it's no longer a daydream, it's a goal, it's something real that you're working towards. While you do want to have a positive attitude, you also need to make your plan realistic. Planning your whole life around, winning the lottery is not realistic. But planning to be healthy and happy should be realistic for anybody.

Portion control.

Portion sizes are huge problem when trying to have a healthy diet. We seem to have completely lost control of portion sizes with pressure from all directions to super-size your meals, have extra helpings, sharing sized packets of crisps and cookies that have exploded into the size of dinner plates. We are silently encouraged at all points to eat far more food that we actually should, so cutting down on excess food can begin by cutting portion sizes.

Eating more food just becomes a habit that we don't even notice, and in the same way, eating less can become a new, healthier habit, and again, you hardly even notice. The plate is still full when you start and you just eat what's on your plate.

10: Use smaller plates. It sounds too simple to work but it does. Plate sizes have matched the rest of us in recent years, they've put on weight, a lot of it! Change your plates for smaller ones and you will automatically have smaller portions. You will still clear your plate, something that most of us have been encouraged to do as children, but you will have eaten far less.

11: Actually measure a portion of food. For instance a healthy portion of breakfast cereal is approximately 40 grams. So measure out 40 g in a bowl that you normally use for your breakfast cereal. You only need to do this once and you will then know how much cereal to put in the bowl, otherwise it's very tempting to either put too little in because you think you're eating less and then you're just hungry or to fill it to the top having no idea how much food you're actually consuming. Repeat the same process with any food that you regularly eat so that you know what a healthy portion actually looks like. If it looks too small on the plate or in the bowl, change to a smaller plate or bowl.

12: Buy smaller packets. Although it is far better to not eat crisps at all, we do live in the real world. So if you are going to eat crisps, make sure that you buy smaller packets. Once you open a packet of crisps you will eat it, so you will naturally eat fewer if you buy smaller packets in the first place.

13: If you do buy large packets of treats such as crisps or popcorn, decant the bag into five or six small storage boxes. In this way you can stick to a small portion by treating yourself to one box rather than eating the whole bag in a single sitting.

14: Don't ban anything. As soon as you decide you mustn't eat :-

    a packet of crisps
    a packet of biscuits
    a chocolate bar
    a burger meal

it is the one thing you'll fixate on and, it might take a while, but you will give in! So don't ban it. Allow yourself a small chocolate bar, try to make it dark chocolate, 85% cocoa if possible it's full of antioxidants and much healthier for you. If you must have crisps, buy smaller bags. Allow yourself the treat but restrict the size. You will get used to it and you'll probably even stop craving the food at all.

15: If you are tempted to cheat - stop and think about who you are cheating on. You. Why would you cheat yourself?

Changing the way you eat

It used to be taken for granted that eating took place at a table. Your meal would be presented on a plate and eaten with a knife and fork.

Time was set for eating – meal times!

But all that has changed.

Now we eat on the go, graze at our desks, grab some fast fool on the way home and generally have lost all sight of actually planning our food intake!

One of the best ways to lose weight without noticing is to actually have meals. You will probably eat more and feel more satisfied when you finish a meal if you actually sit down at a table and eat, rather than grabbing food on the go, or snacking as you sit in front of the TV. That means that you will be less inclined to snack during the rest of the day.

You will also have a better balance of healthy food, a mix of meat and vegetables – in other words, protein, carbohydrates and healthy fat. Of course, vegetarians will have other protein – not meat or fish!

So think about how you actually eat and make some subtle but important changes.

You should also learn to eat mindfully. Eating slowly, taking the time to chew each mouthful, rather than just swallowing it. This will give you the time to think about what you're eating, and to think how good it tastes or otherwise. This will mean that you will learn to make healthier choices simply by actually thinking about the food you are eating.

16: Reinstate meal times. Sit down at a table to eat rather than grazing in front of the TV. It's much too easy to eat far more food than you realise if you just snack all evening. Put the meal on a plate, sit and eat it and feel full.

17: When you're having a meal, put your knife and fork down between mouthfuls. This will automatically slow you down, which is a good thing. If you concentrate on the mouthful that you are actually eating rather than the next forkful you are picking up, you will choose your food more carefully, enjoy the meal more and give your stomach a chance to send signals to the brain when you've actually had enough to eat.

18: In general, try and slow down when you're eating. We've all become used to eating in a rush, on the go, at our desks. Take a meal break and allow your body to digest the fuel you're putting into it.

19: It takes the stomach about 10 minutes to tell the brain that it has had enough food Try chewing your food more thoroughly or take a short break during your meal. If you cram the food down too fast, you can easily eat far more than you need or even actually want, before your brain receives the signal to stop. Then you need the indigestion and heartburn remedies as well.

20: Don't skip meals. Your body needs a steady supply of fuel to keep it going. Skipping meals is not a good way of cutting down on calories and losing weight, it is simply a way of slowing down your metabolism and making you much more likely to reach for a sugar fix. It also means that your body is far more likely to store food as fat to prepare it for the time of famine that it believes is coming.

Breakfast

It's very tempting to think that skipping breakfast is a good way to lose weight. After all, if you missed out one meal altogether it must mean that you eat fewer calories during the day as a total!

But skipping breakfast is the biggest mistake you can make when trying to control your weight.

A good breakfast boosts your metabolism, which means that you will automatically start out each day by having your system ready to burn more calories. Your metabolism naturally slows throughout the day, so in reality, the old saying of breakfast like a king is correct. Having your largest meal at the beginning of the day is a good idea.

The old saying is – breakfast like a king, lunch like a prince, dine like a pauper. In fact, we do the very opposite nowadays. We breakfast as if there is no money and therefore no food in the house, we have fast food snacks for lunch that are often full of empty calories, fat, salt and sugar, and then we dine like a king at the very time of day that the metabolism has slowed down. And to make it even worse we often have wine with the meal, adding more empty calories at the very time of day that the metabolism is at its most sluggish.

A healthy breakfast is protein heavy, to kick start your metabolism and make you feel fuller for longer. So, take a good look at your breakfast habits, they should include good protein foods such as eggs, healthy meat or fish or nuts and seeds. The old fashioned breakfasts that we think of as unhealthy such as omelettes, boiled eggs, scrambled eggs on salmon or kippers are actually a very good way to start the day.

21: Never skip breakfast. If there's one meal you should always eat – it's breakfast. Breaking your fast is the process of telling your metabolism to start working again. It might feel as if skipping breakfast is a good idea but it will simply mean that when you do eat you are more likely to eat more and to store the food as fat.

22: If you tend to eat breakfast cereals, take the time to actually read the nutritional information on the back of the pack. The only way to be able to compare one product with another is to read the information based on the same weight of food, for instance 100g. The information that is printed in large friendly letters on the front of the pack can be based on 30g for one cereal and 50g for another cereal, so it's very difficult to compare like-for-like.

23: Learn to read the nutritional information on food labels, Ingredients are listed in order of quantity, so if sugar is high on the list, it is high in the content of your cereal bowl. You only really need to do this work once, checking the different types of cereal to see which are actually healthier rather than just trusting the advertising promises.

24: Learn to recognise the words that mean sugar! Words ending in 'ose' are normally other words for sugar! Sucrose, fructose, maltose, high fructose corn syrup, dextrose. Names including the word syrup also mean sugar – maple syrup, malt syrup, corn syrup. Sometime labels will include two or more of these in the ingredients list making it appear that 'sugar' is lower down on the list of ingredients, but if you add them together you are eating a very hefty dose of the sweet stuff!

25: So if you do prefer to eat cereal for breakfast, check the levels of sugar very carefully. Some cereals, especially those aimed at children, have so much sugar in them that they are more like sweets. Eating a highly processed, high in sugar cereal will mean that you are hungry again in a very short period of time. Highly processed cereal turns to glucose in the blood very quickly, then add pure glucose (sugar) to the mix and your insulin will be working overtime removing all this glucose and storing it up for later – in fat cells! And to add insult to injury – you will be hungry again and reaching for that mid morning snack. So if you've wondered why you are starving a couple of hours after breakfast – it genuinely isn't your fault!

26: Try to choose a non-sweetened cereal that contains wholegrains that you body will have to work to break down. Cereals such as muesli are a good choice, and if it contains nuts, so much the better. They are a good source of protein.

27: Look for the fibre content in your cereal – high dietary fibre will make your digestive system work more efficiently.

28: If you prefer toast for breakfast, again it is best to choose a whole grain or seeded bread. Try to avoid bagels or white bread, and especially those delicious French breads baked with finely milled white flour. They may taste delicious, but this type of food also breaks down very fast into glucose in the blood stream making you hungry again and reaching for a snack within a couple of hours.

29: The ideal breakfast should be protein rich, because protein will help give you energy, will burn slowly and will keep you feeling full for much longer.

30: Porridge with dried fruits (although not too much – remember that fruit is natural sugar), and cinnamon is a good breakfast, because it is high in protein and porridge oats can help lower your cholesterol levels while the cinnamon can help lower your blood sugar and the dried fruits contain fibre as well as vitamins and nutrients. Make sure you pick natural dried fruit rather than any that has been artificially sweetened.

31: We seem to have spent years being scared of eggs. But in fact, the old adage of go to work on an egg is quite right. A boiled egg, or even two with a slice of whole grain toast is a very healthy start to the day, full of protein.

32: Although it is healthy to add fruit and vegetables to your diet, make sure that your orange juice with breakfast is in a small glass – again, it is a fruit and contains sugar.

33: Swap your fresh orange juice for actual oranges. If you squeeze the juice from five or six oranges you can drink the whole glass at one sitting. But try eating five or six oranges - not as easy! The orange juice contains the same amount of natural sugars but none of the fibre of the whole fruit. Fruit sugar might be natural but it is still sugar, and fibre is vital part of a healthy diet.

34: Check the dietary information on your carton of fruit juice. Many are made from concentrate and contain far more chemicals, water and sugar than actual fruit. You may think you are picking a healthy fruit juice or smoothie, but you are actually adding a significant amount of sugar to your diet.

35: Swap your fruit juice for a vegetable juice and you will automatically cut down on sugar and add nutrients to your diet.

Your Fluid intake

Our bodies are made up of approximately 70% water, and our brains have an even higher percentage. Blood and organs are mainly water and it needs to be replaced to keep us healthy.

We tend to think that we only need to worry about dehydration if we feel thirsty but this is really one of the signs of severe dehydration. Long before you feel thirsty, the body is already suffering from dehydration, which includes feeling tired, irritable, unable to concentrate and suffering frequent headaches.

Many people are in a constant state of dehydration. Signs can include dull skin and the fact that your hair is lacking bounce.

More seriously, it can also include severe fatigue or low heart rate. It can also slow down your digestion and cause constipation.

So it is vital for good health and good body balance to be well hydrated, although you must also be aware that it is possible to drink too much too fast. You should never try to have your entire 2 litre daily supply in one go. Not only would this be very difficult - it would be very dangerous.

36: Drink plenty of water, although not excessive amounts as it can be dangerous. Drink a glass of water half an hour before a meal. You'll want to eat less when you actually do start to eat.

37: Drink water regularly. About 6 to 8 glasses a day (approximately 2 litres). This will keep you hydrated. What we think of as hunger is often really thirst. Once you actually feel thirsty you are already dehydrated, so keeping hydrated will stop you reaching for a snack.

38: When you are having your glass of water, add some ice cubes to it. The body will have to burn a few more calories to warm the icy water in your stomach. It might not be much, but as they say – every little helps!

39: Drinking water between meals will make you less likely to reach for a sugary snack because the water will keep you feeling full.

40: Swap sodas for water. We have become far too used to reaching for a bottle of soda rather than water and it really is just a matter of retraining our taste. Flavour the water with lemon or lime or make a weak solution of juice if you really don't like plain water. Persevere, your taste buds will adapt quite quickly and as a bonus you will be saving money and improving your skin as well as your health – much cheaper than an anti-aging cream.

41: Of course not all your fluids have to be in the form of pure water. Tea is considered to have many health benefits as well as helping to hydrate you. If you take your tea without milk or sugar it is a calorie free drink, unlike a latte which can contain about 100 cal.

Swap your latte for a black tea once a day and you'll be saving yourself. 36,500 calories a year!

42: Green tea contains natural flavonoids which - when combined with the caffeine that also occurs naturally in green tea - is considered to help weight loss and to help you maintain a steady weight once you've reached your target.

43: Research suggests that drinking just 4 cups of black or green tea a day, may have significant health benefits. Just remember to avoid the sugar and biscuits!

44: You can also have some of your fluid intake in the form of fruit or vegetable juices. This is a good way of increasing your vitamin and mineral intake and helping you include enough fruit and vegetables in your diet, but do read the nutrition labels carefully, many fruit juices are full of sugar. Ideally, you should make your own fruit juice, then you will know exactly what you put into it. But even then you must remember that fruit itself is full of natural sugars, so limit the amount that you drink. This also refers to healthy smoothies.

45: Vegetable juice is a healthier alternative to fruit juice and smoothies. A class of carrot juice will provide lots of vitamins and minerals but nowhere near as much sugar.

46: While you are concentrating on all this healthy drinking and hydrating is also very important to remember that alcohol contains a great number of empty calories. Share a bottle of wine with your partner at dinner, and you will be adding approximately 250 cal to your meal total. Try to cut out alcohol altogether while you are in your initial weight loss process. If you feel a social event requires you to have a glass of wine, choose a smaller glass and sip it slowly so that it lasts.

Flavour and your diet

The way food tastes, can have a huge effect on your weight.

We have become so used to salty and overly sweet and fat laden processed foods that our taste buds have been beaten into submission, and the lack of the sense of taste encourages you to eat more than you need, thereby putting on weight.

The good news is that you can help your taste buds recover and learn to enjoy your food again.

When you change your diet from highly processed pre-prepared and fast food back to real food, you will begin to appreciate the natural taste of real food within a few weeks, and once your taste buds have been retrained you will no longer crave high amounts of sugar or salt or greasy foods. In fact, you will discover that not only do you not want them, you actually dislike the taste. And of course this makes it much easier to lose weight.

But don't worry, there are still plenty of healthy ways to get flavour into your food, without piling it full of sugar, salt and unhealthy fats.

It's not a matter of cutting out everything altogether, it is a matter of getting a healthy balance in your diet.

47: If you love cheese (oh I love cheese!) always buy extra mature, strong flavoured cheese, you will use less but get the same cheesy flavour.

48: And grate your cheese, it will go much further and you'll get the flavour and taste with much less actual cheese.

49: When you buy cheese, cut it into small portions - the healthy portion is about the size of a matchbox - then you won't be tempted to use half the block at once. You'll have an easy visual reminder of how much you should use.

50: Add spices to your meals when you're cooking. They will give extra zest and flavour and at the same time will encourage you to take smaller mouthfuls. Hot food is more difficult to handle! This means that your body will send the signals that you've eaten enough on less actual food because you are giving it time for the digestive system to send signals to the brain.

51: As an added bonus, there is research to suggest that spicy food – especially chilli – can actually raise your metabolic rate. Some suggest that this increase can be as much as 8% and can last for three hours after the meal.

52: Add flavour to your food with natural herbs and spices or chillies, rather than chutney or sauce from a bottle. A small dollop of tomato ketchup can contain half a teaspoon of sugar.

53: Adding vinaigrette to your salad or vinegar to your meals can help weight loss by slowing down the absorption of carbohydrates in your body. This means that your sugar levels in the blood will be kept stable, making you feel full for longer and then you're less likely to feel the need for a snack.

54: Cinnamon can also help lower your blood sugar levels, keeping you feeling full for longer. You can add it to recipes, sprinkle it on your porridge or your coffee. But it doesn't work in the form of a cinnamon covered Danish pastry or doughnut!

Learn to love your kitchen

One of the best ways to control your weight is to know what you're actually eating.

Processed foods are made to suit the food industry not the consumer. They are designed to be cost effective (that means cheap to produce), easy to transport, have a long shelf life and create profit. After all they are in business and they have shareholders to keep happy. So the food industry is far more interested in their bottom line than the size of your bottom!

Processed foods contain huge amounts of fat, sugar and salt and at times, very little of nutritional value.

When you cook your own food, you know exactly what you're eating.

The main excuse for many of us in reaching for a micro meal rather than cook proper food - is time. Lack of time! But there are many meals that can be cooked from scratch in about the same amount of time as that tasteless thing that went from freezer to microwave and leaves you feeling hungry.

55: Learn to love eggs. They are a good source of protein, vitamin D, Vitamin A, Vitamin B2 and iodine. They are also versatile and quick to create a meal with. Omelettes, scrambled eggs, eggs Benedict, boiled eggs or fried eggs (with just a spray of healthy oil).

56: Frozen vegetable are a very healthy and simply choice for a meal. Because they are frozen soon after harvesting, they maintain their vitamins and nutrients far better than the 'fresh' vegetable that have travelled many miles and have been in transit, in storage on the supermarket shelves and then your refrigerator for many days, even a week or more. You can make a quick and healthy meal in minutes with some vegetables from your freezer.

57: Set aside a day for cooking and create a batch of meals that you can then freeze, creating your own ready meals. If you make up a large pan of vegetables in tomato sauce it can be frozen into individual containers and then made into meals by simply thawing, heating and adding rice, pasta, new potatoes and meat or fish of your choice.

58: Choose tomato based sauces rather than rich cream or cheese sauce. The tomato sauce contains far less fat and is rich in antioxidants. It is said to help reduce the risk of macular degeneration and cataracts, and help maintain mental function as we age as well as helping protect our immune system. And cooking the tomatoes increases the health benefits. It also contains far less fat and fewer calories that a cheesy sauce.

59: When you are cooking, try to avoid coconut milk in your recipes. It is very high in fat and should be kept as an occasional treat rather than an everyday ingredient.

60: Choose cold pressed oils such as olive oil or cold pressed rape seed oil rather than vegetable oils for your cooking. They are healthier and taste better.

61: Invest in an oil spray and use this rather than pouring oils straight from a bottle into your pan, you will automatically add a lot less oil to your cooking.

62: Try other cooking methods in the kitchen. Grill, poach or steam fish and chicken rather than frying and if you can't do without the Sunday roast, use a rack to cook it on, allowing the fat to drain into the roasting pan rather than transferring to your plate.

63: Reduce the amount of red meat in your diet and choose cuts that have a lower fat content. Cut down gradually rather than going cold turkey – pardon the pun! If you normally eat red meat three times a week, make it twice a week and then cut it back to a special treat once a week. Feeling deprived is a sure way to failure when you're trying to make long term changes in your eating plan.

64: Replace your red meat with chicken and remove the skin as this will automatically make it a lower fat meal.

65: And of course you can add a lot of extra exercise to your routine by spending some time in the kitchen. Check out my book '101 ways to exercise without noticing' for more ideas.

Food to avoid

Although it is not a good idea to ban any favourite food in your diet, there are certainly foods that you should avoid when you're going around the supermarket.

It's also a good idea to put a little more thought into how you actually shop for food. Rushing around the supermarket when you're tired and hungry and short of time is a sure fire way to pile your trolley with all the wrong choices.

Make time for shopping. Make sure you've eaten before you go. Have a list prepared so you know what you're looking for and give yourself time to read the labels and make the right choices.

And don't say that you haven't got the time – make the time!

You're worth some investment in time and as you begin to lose the weight and feel healthier you'll be able to do so much more with your time because you won't be feeling tired and depressed.

So spend some time making our your list and then shop with that list rather than just grabbing whatever is on the shelf and calling out to you as you pass.

If you find you cannot resist sugary popcorn, potato chips, large bars of chocolate or double cream, then it's best to avoid the temptation by not actually having your particular poison in the cupboard at home where it is easy to reach for.

Save your particular weakness for a special occasion or only have it when you're eating out - and that does not include eating lunch out everyday!

There are other foods and food types that you should simply avoid altogether.

66: Avoid meals that claim to be low-fat. If you read the nutritional information of a normal version and a low-fat version, you will normally find that there is very little difference in the amount of fat but much more sugar and salt in the low-fat version, the flavour has to come from somewhere.

67: Avoid foods that are labelled as healthy. The label is simply a marketing strategy, and very rarely has any actual nutritional value. Many diet foods can be loaded with salt, otherwise labelled as sodium. For instance, a low-fat cottage cheese could have more salt than a packet of potato chips.

68: Avoid fat free salad dressings, they are often loaded with sugar to compensate for the lower fat levels. A fat free honey and mustard dressing could have as much as 8 grams of sugar in a couple of tablespoons. Choose a vinaigrette dressing instead, it will have far less sugar and vinaigrette can help slow down the absorption of carbohydrates, leaving you feeling full for longer.

69: In fact, avoid foods that are labelled low fat altogether. The supermarkets are loaded with healthy looking packages of cookies, yoghurts, cakes, salad dressings, and all sorts of other treats and meals labelled low fat, but they are often full of sugars, sweeteners, salt and other unpronounceable ingredients that everyone should avoid. Instead of filling yourself up on fattening 'healthy' treats, choose real food, and if you can't resist cookies and biscuits, treat yourself to good quality versions now and again. You will appreciate them more if you eat far less.

70: Avoid processed meat when you're filling up your shopping trolley. Research shows that meats that have been preserved by salting, curing or smoking, contain chemicals that have been linked to various types of cancer. They also tend to include large amounts of salt and fat and very little in the way of nutritional goodness. Choose chicken pieces to add to your meal rather than hot dogs or luncheon meat.

71: Avoid frozen meals, they might seem like an easy answer but they are not. They are often full of salt and sugar. Even if they are labelled as low-fat meals, they are still a very bad choice. Even worse when you look more closely at the relatively low calorie counts, printed in big friendly letters on the front of the pack, it often refers to a serving of half the pack when they are clearly only suitable as a meal for one.

72: Avoid doughnuts! They are probably one of the unhealthiest foods ever devised, often containing trans fats, sugar and highly refined flour, which can add up to about 300 empty calories and a feeling of hunger soon after you've eaten one, that's why people can never stop at one.

73: Avoid soda. In the West we have developed an addiction to soda, which is understandable, because an average can of soda can contain up to 10 teaspoons of sugar, and sugar is highly addictive. The more you drink, the more you want to drink.

74: Avoid diet soda. Although diet soda doesn't contain the sugars, they are loaded with artificial sweeteners instead and research has shown that when the body consumes something sweet without the carbohydrates that would normally come with sugar, it still craves the carbohydrates, and you are more likely to reach for a sugary snack. There is also research to show that when you drink soda with Zero calories you feel virtuous, and that you can afford to eat some calories in the form of - you guessed it - a sugary snack!

75: Avoid healthy smoothies and fruit juices. They are marketed as being full of goodness and giving you one or two portions of fresh fruit, making it an easy way to increase the portions of fresh fruit and vegetables that you are getting in your diet each day. But when you eat an orange you are getting a mixture of the natural fruit sugars with fibre, vitamins and nutrients. Most people could only eat one or two oranges, but if you have a glass of orange juice, you will be consuming the juice of up to 6 oranges, with all of the fruit sugars that come with six oranges, and none of the fibre. To make it worse most of the smoothies and fruit juices available are made from fruit concentrate rather than fresh fruit.

Foods to choose.

There are some foods that will actually help improve your weight loss when you add them to your diet. We tend to think of dieting simply as cutting out food, either cutting out bad food or cutting down on food consumption altogether.

Of course, it is true that in order to lose weight you need to reduce the number of calories you eat, but you can also add some foods to your diet which will help your metabolism work more efficiently and therefore helps you lose weight. A healthy diet often includes more food than the unhealthy diet you're replacing. Fewer calories but more food, more vitamins, nutrients and fibre which will make the digestion and your whole body work more efficiently and make you feel healthier as well as helping you lose weight.

You should try adding these foods to your everyday diet to help you lose weight without having to feel hungry - it will never work if you feel hungry on a diet, suffering might be good for the soul according to some people, but it certainly isn't good when you're wanting to lose weight!

76: Add eggs to your menu. We seem to have been frightened of eggs for years, fearing that they are bad for cholesterol or just unhealthy altogether, but in fact, they are a very healthy part of the diet. They are full of protein, which will make you feel full for much longer after your meal. Research has shown that someone who chooses two scrambled eggs with whole grain toast for breakfast, rather than a bagel or white toast, actually eats less for the rest of the day.

77: Add beans to your menu. Again, beans are full of protein which will help you feel fuller for longer. There is also research to show that beans contain a digestive hormone that will naturally suppress your appetite. They are also full of fibre, which again will keep you feeling full and there is some research to show that they will help keep blood sugar levels even, which is not only good for those with diabetes but for everyone, because if your blood sugar levels are kept even, you will not suffer from the spikes in hunger which lead you to grabbing a sugar snack.

78: Start your meal with a nice salad of greens, tomatoes and peppers, rather than a slice of garlic bread. The salad with vinaigrette dressing, rather than a rich creamy dressing, will mean that you will eat less of your main course. A nice fresh salad is also a very good way to improve your intake of vitamins and nutrients.

79: Swap your coffee for green tea. Tea, especially green tea is full of antioxidants, which are believed to help speed up your metabolism and therefore your fat burning rate. Without milk or sugar, tea is also a Zero calorie drink.

80: Include more calcium in your diet. We tend to think of calcium deficiency as being linked to osteoporosis, which of course it is. But calcium has a far larger role to play in the body, and many of us simply don't have enough calcium in our diets. There have been research projects that have shown that when there are two groups on the same diet, and one group has added calcium, (and therefore added calories), it is that group, who have a higher weight loss. They also have a greater loss of belly fat, considered the most important area to lose fat from. Try to include three servings of calcium in your daily diet, such as a glass of milk or a natural yoghurt. The obvious choices are milk and yoghurt and other dairy products, but you can also get calcium from leafy vegetables, prunes and figs.

81: Use low-fat plain yoghurt instead of mayonnaise as a topping for a baked potato, a salad dressing or in making your own dip.

82: To make a really healthy snack, make your own dip with low-fat yoghurt by adding some garlic and herbs, cayenne pepper or cinnamon. There are many recipes for healthy yoghurt dips, so you can create the ones you like. Serve them with sticks of raw carrot, slices of cucumbers and peppers, and small tomatoes, and you will have a very healthy, filling and tasty alternative to your normal chips and dips.

83: Choose fruits, rather than potato chips and chocolate bars as a snack. They are healthier and include vitamins and nutrients, rather than fats and unpronounceable ingredients. Pears and apples are a very good source of fibre, which will help keep you feeling full for longer and although grapes are full of antioxidants, they are also full of natural fruit sugars, so you should only have a handful a day.

84: Learn to love soup. Although it may sound strange, research has shown that there is a difference between eating a plate of food and a glass of water or eating the food and water blended together in a soup. Eating the soup keeps you feeling full for longer and therefore less likely to reach for more food. Vegetable soup is best because it is naturally lower in calories.

85: Not only is extra virgin olive oil a healthy monounsaturated fat, research shows that even the aroma of olive oil can make you feel fuller. Make sure that you are buying good quality, genuine, extra virgin olive oil, rather than a cheap substitute. It is perfect drizzled over salads or pasta or mixed with balsamic vinegar to make a dressing. You can also use it Italian style as a dip for your bread rather than using butter or spread.

86: Add cinnamon to your breakfast oatmeal or to some of your recipes - not cinnamon buns! Cinnamon is considered to help keep your blood sugar levels in control and therefore help reduce the spikes in insulin, which can make you feel hungry.

87: Add nuts to your diet. Many people avoid nuts because they are high in calories and fat, but it is unsaturated fat, which is healthier for us. Research has shown that people who snack on a handful of nuts tend to eat less when they sit down for a meal. And nuts are full of protein and nutrients. Walnuts and Brazil nuts are rich in omega-3 fatty acids, although Brazil nuts are also very high in selenium, so you should probably only eat one or two a day. Obviously, you should choose unsalted nuts, and preferably raw rather than ones roasted in oil or covered in sugar. Cashew nuts are high in antioxidants, peanuts are a very good source of protein, and almonds are high in vitamins D and vitamin B2.

88: Adding seeds to your diet is another way of boosting your energy and keeping you feeling full. Add pumpkin seeds, sesame, sunflower or flax seeds to your salads or use them as a healthy snack. When you are adding nuts or seeds to your diet, do remember that you can have too much of a good thing! A handful a day is a good way to get the nutritional benefits, and keep hunger at bay.

89: Prawns are a rich source of many vitamins and minerals, as well as being a good source of protein, but they are also very low in calories and they don't absorb too much oil in the cooking process. All of this makes them a healthier choice to add to your pasta, salad or stirfry than chicken or beef.

90: Learn to love chilli. For those of us who love hot food, the good news is that the chemicals in chillies can help boost the body's ability to burn fat, by stimulating the natural process of turning some of the food we are eating to heat, allowing the calories to be burnt, rather than stored as fat.

91: Eating fresh vegetables is not only a good source of vitamins and minerals, is also a very good source of fibre. Root vegetables such as carrots and parsnips in particular, are very high in fibre, which will help your digestive system and keep you feeling full for longer. Try eating raw carrot sticks as a snack or making a tasty vegetable juice.

92: Make sure that you include plenty of leafy green vegetables in your diet, such as spinach, broccoli and cabbage. Apart from being full of vitamins and minerals, they are also very filling, and very low in calories and meaning you can eat almost as much as you want.

Healthy snacking.

Losing weight should not ever be about suffering hunger and denying yourself. Although many diets do seem to be all about self-denial, in reality, they don't work.

Nutritionally they are a very bad idea, because although you may lose weight on a crash diet you will almost certainly can put it straight back on again as soon as you start eating normally.

They are also bad idea because they set you up to fail. You may have the willpower to put up with the hunger and the boredom for a few days. But then you will fall off the wagon, feel as if you are a terrible failure, console yourself with a huge bag of potato chips or a tub of ice cream and then just forget about the diet thing altogether.

In order to have a successful weight loss program that you will stick to, you need to avoid hunger. You also need to avoid the quick fix chocolate bars, cookies and doughnuts that are so easily to hand, the empty calories that you find yourself eating without even realising it.

Make sure that you have a ready supply of healthy snacks that will help you reach your weight goal and keep there once you've lost the weight. They have to be available, easy and convenient otherwise the vending machine will win.

Healthy snacking will help you eat less at mealtimes, because you won't be overwhelmed with hunger and then eat more than you need to feel full.

A snack should be about 150 to 200 calories and be enough to make you feel satisfied. If it isn't, you'll still reach for a chocolate bar out of the vending machine as you pass it.

Prepare snacks in advance and keep them handy in the fridge so that they are easy to reach for when you're busy and hungry. Healthy snacking has to be as easy as unhealthy snacking otherwise the unhealthy, fattening snacks will win the day.

93: Keep a supply of apples around. An apple is fine to eat on its own, but if you have a little more time you can also make a very simple small snack salad by chopping the apple and mixing it with some chopped walnuts, lettuce and celery and finishing it off with a vinaigrette dressing

94: A handful of nuts is a great snack. Although they contain high levels of fat, it's the healthy fats, and they are full of protein, which will help keep you feeling full and mean that you eat less once you get to your main meal.

95: Create a rich and creamy snack with half an avocado and some cottage cheese. Simply remove the pit from the centre of the avocado and fill it with plain, cottage cheese. You'll get a good serving of protein and fibre for about 200 cal.

96: Mix a small can of tuna in spring water, with some black pepper and chopped red onion. Serve on a couple of rye crackers for a very satisfying snack, full of protein and healthy omega-3 oils.

97: Make a small salad with lentils, chopped celery, red onion, cherry tomatoes and watercress and top off with a vinaigrette dressing, adding black pepper to taste.

98: Add some pomegranate seeds to a pot of natural yoghurt. They not only tastes delicious, the pomegranate seeds are a good source of vitamins C and K are low in calories and contained dietary fibre.

99: Carry a small serving, about 1 ounce, of dried fruit and cashew nuts or almonds with you. If you get the munchies while you're out and about this will save you reaching for the nearest chocolate bar or vending machine.

100: As long as you avoid the sweet sugary or the greasy buttery versions, popcorn is an excellent snack. A cup of plain popcorn only contains about 30 cal, and it also has fibre and is 100% whole grain, which means it contains antioxidants. If you want to add some flavour try drizzling some olive oil over it once it's cooked, or sprinkling some sea salt or pepper - adding salt to the surface of food, rather than in the cooking process means that you get much more taste with far less salt. If you prefer a spicy snack, add paprika or chilli powder. If you prefer a sweeter taste, try ground cinnamon or grated nutmeg.

101: And saving the best till last - for everyone who loves chocolate - the good news is that chocolate can be good for you. It has to be dark chocolate, the darker the better, at least 70% cocoa, preferably 85% cocoa.

There has been quite a lot of research recently that shows that those who eat good quality dark chocolate are slimmer than those who don't eat chocolate at all. Cacao is a rich source of flavonoids, an important antioxidant and has also been shown to have an effect on our moods and hunger cravings, stabilising moods and helping to boost positive feeling, which can help you ward off the stress and depression that can defeat your willpower and leave you heading for the fridge. Although, dark chocolate is only a small part of a successful healthy eating plan, it is a very tasty part. Of course, moderation in all things, you should restrict yourself to about 40 grams of strong, dark chocolate a day.

I hope you find these ideas useful. Healthy eating and making healthier food choices is a habit.

We have been brainwashed into making unhealthy choices and creating unhealthy, fattening habits even when we think we're making the right choices by choosing low fat foods, diet bars, diet sodas and 'healthy' smoothies.

When that is added to the groaning shelves of cookies, cakes, breads, calorie heavy meals and then a caramel macchiato weighing in at almost 400 calories or a rich hot chocolate at almost 700 calories with a chocolate chip cookie adding another 500 calories, it's hardly surprising that we have just lost the plot!

But remember, good habits are just as easy to create as bad habits, and you often just need a bit of active rethinking to help you swap those bad habits for good!

About the Author

Marianne Duvall's passion in life is showing people how to make it easy to live a healthier life through nutrition and fitness – making small changes in everyday life that can make big changes in health and wellbeing.

She has studied how to rebalance modern life to allow space for good nutrition and activity as part of everyday life rather than an expensive and time consuming extra.

She believes that healthy living should be how we live, part of everyday life rather than an afterthought. Something so natural that we don't even think about it, we just do it.

She has developed her ideas over the years working with those living with chronic illnesses such as M.E./CFS, fibromyalgia or diabetes, developing plans that help people live successfully with these illnesses.

Her motto is 'Live Life'